Copyright © 2020 by Eric Goldinger

All rights reserved. This book or any portion thereof may not be reproduced or used in any manner whatsoever without the express written permission of the publisher except for the use of brief quotations in a book review.

DISCLAIMER

By reading this disclaimer, you fully accept the terms of this disclaimer. If you are not in agreement with this disclaimer, please do not order or read this book. The content of this book is provided for information and educational purposes only. Kindly do not interpret this book or its content for a medication or product. This is only a book guide.

Thanks

61+ AMAZING USES AND BENEFITS OF HYDROGEN PEROXIDE
BY ERIC GOLDINGER

Table of Contents

INTRODUCTION 6

   Features of Hydrogen Peroxide 8

   Brief History of Discovery 14

   Properties of Hydrogen Peroxide 16

   The Chemical Formula and Structure of Hydrogen Peroxide 18

   Preparation of Hydrogen Peroxide 19

   Grades of Hydrogen Peroxide 21

   Forms of Hydrogen Peroxide 22

   Highlights about Hydrogen Peroxide 25

USES & BENEFITS OF HYDROGEN PEROXIDE 27

   Medicinal Uses of Hydrogen Peroxide 27

      Cleaning Contact Lenses 27

      Treat Sinus Infection 28

      Ease a Sore Throat 30

      Appease Dry Skin 30

      Clean and Disinfect Small Cuts 31

      Treat Acne 31

      Treat Canker Sores 32

      Get Rid of Bad Breath with a Peroxide Mouth Rinse 33

      Battle Foot Fungus 34

      Treat Nail Fungus 34

- Treat Colds 35
- Treat Ear Infections 35
- Ear Wax Removal 36
- Treat Toothache 37
- Detoxifying Bath 38
- Treating Yeast Infections 40
- Teeth Whitener 42
- Use as a Toothpaste 43
- Disinfect Toothbrush 43
- Treatment for Gum Disease 45

Beauty Used of Hydrogen Peroxide 46
- Use as Deodorant 46
- Clean Makeup Brushes 47
- Whiten Your Nails 48
- Cover Darker Roots 48
- Lighten the Hair 49
- Soften Corns and Calluses on Your Feet 49
- House Cleaning Uses of Hydrogen Peroxide 50
- Disinfecting Countertops 51
- Whiten Grout 51
- Cleaning the Mirrors 52
- Clean Toilet 52
- Clean Bathroom Tiles 54

61+ AMAZING USES AND BENEFITS OF HYDROGEN PEROXIDE
BY ERIC GOLDINGER

Kills Mold 55

Remove Stains from Marble 55

Cleaning Windows 56

Water Sanitation 57

Clean Children's Toys 59

Cleaning Humidifier or Dehumidifier 59

Kitchen Uses of Hydrogen Peroxide 60

Clean Your Cutting Boards 60

Add It to Your Dishwasher 61

Disinfect the Inside of Your Cooler with Peroxide 61

Sanitize Your Reusable Bags 62

Removes Stubborn Caked-On Food 62

Disinfect Your Sponges and Dishrags 63

Clean Your Fruits and Vegetables 64

Keeping Fruits and Vegetables Fresh 64

Keeping Salad Fresh 65

Cleaning the Fridge 65

Grow Mushrooms in Refrigerator 66

Disinfect Kid's Lunchboxes 66

Hydrogen Peroxide usage in the Laundry Room 67

Brighten Curtains and Table Cloths 68

Wash Your Shower Curtains 69

Remove Tough Stains from White Clothing 69

61+ AMAZING USES AND BENEFITS OF HYDROGEN PEROXIDE
BY ERIC GOLDINGER

- Clean Rugs, Carpet and Mattress 70
- Remove Odors from Clothes and Carpet 71
- Hydrogen Peroxide usage in Gardening 72
  - Increase Plant Growth with Hydrogen Peroxide 72
  - Get Rid of Weeds 73
  - Cleaning Compost Buckets 73
  - Eliminate Algae from Your Aquarium 74
- Hydrogen Peroxide for Animal and Pet Care 75
  - Kill Mites 75
  - Help Transport Fish 75
  - Treat Animal Wounds 75
  - Induce Vomiting to Save Your Pet's Life 76
  - Remove Skunk Odors 76
- Hydrogen Peroxide Side Effects 77
- How and Where to Buy Hydrogen Peroxide 78
- WARNING 79

61+ AMAZING USES AND BENEFITS OF HYDROGEN PEROXIDE
BY ERIC GOLDINGER

INTRODUCTION

Hydrogen Peroxide is an exceptional home remedy that addresses a number of health-related conditions. There are many advantages to H2O therapy. It eliminates infection, reduces pain, detoxifies the body and serves various purposes both inside and outside the home. It is no surprise that hydrogen peroxide is considered a "super miraculous product."

As of now, if you don't have it in your home. Truth be told, this is one of the cheapest, most handy family unit supplies. Also, you'd be amazed at exactly how many ways you can use it for cleaning, and that's just the tip of the iceberg. I'm going to share with you a huge amount of amazing hydrogen peroxide versatility.

Hydrogen peroxide, a chemical that appears as a colorless liquid, is used in a wide range of cleaning and personal care products, including hair dyes and bleaches, toothpaste and mouthwashes, bathroom cleaners and laundry stain removers. Hydrogen peroxide can also be found in over-the-counter (OTC) first aid antiseptics, and it is used as a bleaching agent in some food products. It has other consumer and industrial uses as well, including water treatment.

Hydrogen peroxide is made of hydrogen and oxygen (H2O2). It's a natural disinfectant that bubbles when it comes into contact with an enzyme called catalase. Catalase is found in most cells including blood cells and some bacteria. However, it is not found on the surface of human skin, which is why hydrogen peroxide only bubbles on broken skin. Those bubbles are a reaction that releases oxygen gas.

Hydrogen peroxide has a shelf life of approximately six months after it is opened. The bottle should be stored in a cool, dark place, which is why hydrogen peroxide is normally packaged in a brown bottle. Light and heat can break the compound down, so your bathroom's medicine cabinet may actually not be the best place for it.

Expired hydrogen peroxide isn't harmful, but it won't necessarily be effective. Luckily, there is an easy test to see if your bottle is still good. Just pour a little bit down the bathroom sink the solution should react with the metal drain and bubble. If it doesn't, that means it's time for a new bottle.

Features of Hydrogen Peroxide

Activeness in Oral Care Products

Hydrogen peroxide is an oxidizing agent incorporated in certain mouthwashes (1.5%) recommended for short-term use to eradicate anaerobic bacteria found in conditions such as necrotizing ulcerative gingivitis or periodontitis. It can also have a mechanical cleaning effect as it produces oxygen bubbles when it comes into contact with tissues and debris.

Chemiluminescence

Hydrogen peroxide is produced in various enzymatic reactions, and its determination is the basis for a number of assay methods. A direct ECL method is based on the use of tantalum or zirconium electrodes covered with a terbium (III)-doped oxide layer. Light with the typical emission spectrum of terbium (III) is emitted from the surface of the electrode in the presence of hydrogen peroxide.

In indirect ECL methods, hydrogen peroxide is electrolytically generated by a negatively biased glass carbon or gold electrode and detected by chemiluminescence of, e.g., luminosity. Hydrogen peroxide is transported by liquid flow to the chemiluminescent reagent, and during this time the sample molecules acting as a catalyst are partially decomposed. For example, the sample could be heme components that effectively catalyze the decomposition of hydrogen peroxide.

Sterilization of Flexible Endoscopes

Hydrogen peroxide liquid has been used as an antimicrobial since the beginning of the 20th century; however, for sterilization, concentrations and contact time are too high to be of use. A significantly lower concentration of hydrogen peroxide is needed in the gas. Hydrogen peroxide gas may also be used in a condensed or non-condensed form and each method needs to be evaluated in its own right.

Laundry

Hydrogen peroxide is one of the most common agents of bleaching. Positive aspects of hydrogen peroxide include the fact that it is highly environmentally friendly (decomposes to O2 and H2O), colorless and non-corrosive. It is a very selective bleaching agent because it causes less damage to textile fiber compared to many bleaching systems and tends to be less aggressive to tissue dyes, detergent enzymes and optical brighteners. One drawback is that for hydrogen peroxide to be effective, alkaline conditions and temperatures of around 50 ° C or more are needed. Perhydroxyl anion (HO−2) is thought to be an active bleaching species.

The most stable form of hydrogen peroxide is its dissociated form of the peracid (HOOH, pKa = 11.6), and as a result, most commercial products containing free hydrogen peroxide are formulated at acidic pH. In addition, decomposition of hydrogen peroxide can also occur readily in the presence of certain transition metal ions such as Fe, Mn or Cu.

Likewise, other easily oxidisable substances may promote wasteful hydrogen peroxide decomposition, as can catalase, an enzyme which is almost invariably present on garments worn in contact with the skin, and which catalysis the dismutation of hydrogen peroxide. In an attempt to reduce such problems, especially with respect to the transition-metal catalyzed route, hydrogen peroxide or its derivatives is in most commercial applications formulated together with additives such as transition-metal-chelating agents.

Biocides: Peroxygen Compounds

Inorganic peroxides and peroxy acids can be effective biocides whether they be inorganic peroxides or organic peroxy-compounds.

Inorganic Peroxides

Hydrogen peroxide has good microbial properties, particularly at elevated temperatures. The product itself has been used as a disinfectant in concentrations ranging from 1 to 50%. It is a very reactive material and should not be mixed with other chemicals. Solid products such as sodium percarbonate or sodium perborate release hydrogen peroxide when dissolved in water and are used in powder detergents.

Peroxy Acids

Peracetic acid is the predominant product in this class of peroxy compounds. Commercial products are an equilibrium mixture of hydrogen peroxide, acetic acid, water and peracetic acid. These products have an extremely broad spectrum of antimicrobial activity, including effectiveness against spores, have rapid action and some tolerance to soiling. Environmental acceptability has led to increased use, although the pungent odour of concentrated products and corrosivity to the skin and some metals can be a disadvantage. Other peracids used include peroctanoic acid and magnesium mono-peroxyphthalate.

Brief History of Discovery

In 1799, Alexander Von Humboldt synthesized barium peroxide, one of the first synthetic peroxides, as a by-product of his attempts to decompose air. After 19 years, louise Jacques Thenard stated that this compound could be used for the preparation of a previously unknown compound. He described it as eauoxgenee (French:

Oxygenated Water) which came to be known as Hydrogen Peroxide. And advanced version of Thenard's method was followed from the end of 19th century until the middle of the 20th century. In 1811, Thenard and Joseph Louis Gay-Lussac synthesized sodium peroxide. Pure Hydrogen Peroxide was initially believed to be unstable since early experiments to separate it from the water, which is present synthesis, all failed. This instability was present owing to traces of impurities (transition-metal salts). These impurities catalyze the decomposition of the hydrogen peroxide. Richard Wolfenstein first obtained pure hydrogen peroxide in 1894. He produced it by vacuum distillation.

Properties of Hydrogen Peroxide

- It is almost colorless (very pale blue) in a pure state.

- Its boiling point has been extrapolated at a temperature as high as 150.2C which is almost 50C higher than the boiling point of water

- The melting point of hydrogen peroxide is -0.43C

- It forms a homogenous mixture in all proportion and form hydrates.

- 34.0147g/mol is the molar mass of hydrogen peroxide

- It has a slightly sharp odor

- Its density is 1.11g/cc in aqueous solution and 1.450 g/cc in its pure form

- Hydrogen peroxide is soluble in ether, alcohol but insoluble in petroleum ether.

- It is miscible in water, i.e. it forms a homogeneous solution when mixed with water

- It is acidic in nature.

- H_2O_2 is a very strong oxidizing agent. It gives up one oxygen atom and forms water as a byproduct

$$PbS + 4H_2O_2 \rightarrow PbSO_4 + 4H_2O \text{ (in acidic medium)}$$

$$2Fe + H_2O_2 \rightarrow 2Fe + 2OH \text{ (in basic medium)}$$

- It can also act as a reducing agent if one of the reactants is a stronger oxidizing agent than hydrogen peroxide itself.

$$HOCl + H_2O_2 \rightarrow H_3O + Cl + O_2 \text{ (in acidic medium)}$$

$$I_2 + H_2O_2 + 2OH \rightarrow 2I + 2H_2O + O_2$$

The Chemical Formula and Structure of Hydrogen Peroxide

Hydrogen peroxide has the chemical formula H_2O_2. Its molecular formula is H_2O_2 and its molar mass is 34.0147 g mol-1. Hydrogen peroxide the simplest peroxide (compound with O-O bond) and its structure is H-O-O-H, thus hydrogen peroxide is called as "oxygenated water" because it is a water molecule with one more oxygen atom. The H_2O_2 is a nonplanar molecule with the O-O bond in a plane and the two hydrogen atoms are positioned in "V". This structure has a C2 symmetry axis and it is known as "open book geometry". Its chemical structure can be written as below.

$$\begin{array}{c} H \\ \diagdown \\ O-O \\ \diagdown \\ H \end{array}$$

61+ AMAZING USES AND BENEFITS OF HYDROGEN PEROXIDE
BY ERIC GOLDINGER

If you look at the dot diagram of H2O2 you will see the O-O bond. And you will see that both oxygen atoms have two pairs of unbound electrons each. This brings into effect the valence shell electron repulsion theory.

The hydrogen atoms will repel the unbonded electrons of oxygen. This gives a bent molecular shape. And it has a bod angel of 109.5° in its crystal form (solid state) this angel reduces due to hydrogen bonding within the molecules being formed.

Preparation of Hydrogen Peroxide

1) From Barium Peroxide

This is a method for laboratory preparation of Hydrogen Peroxide. Hydrated Barium Peroxide must be used, anhydrous barium peroxide will form a protective layer and not react with the sulphuric acid. The resulting H2O2 is a 5% concentrate solution.

$$BaO_2 \cdot 8H_2O + H_2SO_4 \rightarrow BaSO_4 + H_2O_2 + 8H_2O$$

2) From Sodium Peroxide

Here too we will use a dilute solution of Sulphuric Acid and gradually dissolve sodium peroxide in it. As you know H2O2 is explosive at high temperatures, so we use cold sulphuric acid. On reacting these two we get crystals of Sodium Sulphide and a 30% solution of hydrogen peroxide. We can perform vacuum distillation on the said solution to get pure hydrogen peroxide

$$Na_2O_2 + H_2SO_4 \rightarrow Na_2SO_4 + H_2O_2 \text{ (30\%)}$$

Hydrogen peroxide is produced in a five-step process:

Hydrogenation → Oxidation → Extraction → Drying/reversion → Distillation, according to the following (simplified) reaction: $H_2 + O_2 \rightarrow H_2O_2$

Grades of Hydrogen Peroxide

- Pharmaceutical Grade (usually 3%) This can be purchased at the drugstore and is used for cleaning wounds and as a general household disinfectant. This grade will generally contain stabilizers.
- Beautician Grade (3 to 12%) For use as hair bleach and contains stabilizers.
- Reagent Grade (usually 30%) Used in scientific experiments, also contains stabilizers.
- Electronic Grade (usually 30% to 35%) Used to clean electronic equipment. Contains stabilizers.
- Technical Grade (usually 35%) Contains a small amount of phosphorus to neutralize any chlorine in the water it is combined with.
- Food Grade (usually 35%) This is used in many food preparation processes, for

instance, in aseptic packaging and bleaching some processed foods.

- 90% Hydrogen Peroxide Used by the military as a source of oxygen, at Cape Canaveral and as rocket fuel

Forms of Hydrogen Peroxide

Simple Hydrogen Peroxide

Most hydrogen peroxide applications require its easy injection into the water stream without the need for additional chemicals or equipment. These involve the regulation of biogrowth (slime), the provision of supplementary oxygen, the removal of FOG and chlorine residues, and the oxidation of sulfides / sulphites, metals and other easy-to-oxidize BOD / COD materials. Activation of H_2O_2 in such applications can be influenced by pH, temperature, and/or reaction time adjustment / control.

Catalytic Hydrogen Peroxide

The more difficult-to-oxidize contaminants that involve the activation of hydrogen peroxide with catalysts such as iron, copper, manganese or other metal transition compounds. These catalysts can also be used to accelerate H_2O_2 reactions that would otherwise take hours or days to complete. Catalysis of H_2O_2 can occur either in solution (using soluble catalysts) or in packed columns (using solid catalysts).

Solution Catalysis

The most widely used solution catalyst is iron, which is referred to as Fenton's Reagent when used with H_2O_2. The reaction requires a slightly acidic pH and results in the formation of highly reactive hydroxyl radicals (.OH) capable of destroying most organic pollutants. Another solution catalyst is copper, which is also used to dissolve cyanide.

Many metals also display catalytic activity with H2O2 and can be used to selectively kill particular pollutants.

Packed Column Catalysis

Solid catalysts remove the need to add soluble metals to the waste stream and may have greater versatility in terms of reaction levels, selectivity and the need for pH adjustment. This is an important area of research and a number of new developments are underway for a variety of applications.

Advanced Oxidation Processes (AOP's)

AOPs are the latest advances in hydrogen peroxide technology and are broadly described as processes that produce highly reactive oxygen radicals without the addition of metal catalysts. Usually, this means the combination of H2O2 with ozone or ultraviolet radiation. The effect is the complete on-site degradation of even refractory organic goods without the generation of sludge or residues. This technology is commonly used to treat polluted groundwater, to purify and clean drinking water and waste water, and to remove trace organics in industrial effluents.

Highlights about Hydrogen Peroxide

• 3.5% is considered pharmaceutical grade, and you can purchase it in local drugstores and grocery stores. It's the most favorite type and the one that is most familiar. It contains a variety of stabilizers, including acetanilide, sodium stannate, phenol, and tetrasodium phosphate and even though it's high in oxygen, it's not intended for internal use.

• 6% is known as beautician grade and is used in beauty salons to color hair.

- 30% is the reagent grade, used for a variety of scientific experiments. It also contains some stabilizers and is not intended for internal use.

- 30- to 32% is an electronic grade, and it's mainly used to clean electronic parts.

- 35% is known as technical grade and is more concentrated than the reagent grade. It differs slightly due to the added phosphorus that is used to help neutralize any chlorine found in the water that is used to dilute it.

- 35% is also known as food-grade hydrogen peroxide. It sees use in the production process of cheese, whey-containing products, and eggs. 35% is also common in products like fruit juices and milk stored in aseptic packages. 35% is the only grade of hydrogen peroxide you can use internally.

- 90% grade hydrogen peroxide sees use in rocket fuel as an oxygen source.

USES & BENEFITS OF HYDROGEN PEROXIDE

Amazing Medicinal, Beauty and Household Uses of Hydrogen Peroxide

Hydrogen peroxide, or H2O2, is a low-cost, handy household product that can be used for cleaning, healing, hygiene and more. You may already have a bottle of it in your house, but if you don't, you can buy it at any drug store or grocery store for a couple of dollars.

Medicinal Uses of Hydrogen Peroxide

Cleaning Contact Lenses

If you wear contact lenses, you know that over time, they can accumulate a buildup of proteins. While you probably use a commercial contact lens cleaner to get rid of these proteins, a cheaper alternative is to use hydrogen peroxide. You can clean contact lenses with 3% hydrogen peroxide by letting them soak for a few hours. This is supposed to break up the protein buildup.

Treat Sinus Infection

A sinus is a membranous cavity present in the bones of the nose, eyes, and cheeks. The membranes function as a filter for germs by producing mucus. Sometimes, these cavities can become clogged or congested, causing an inflammatory response. This can cause pain in your forehead and along your cheeks and nose.

In most cases, sinusitis (inflammation in the sinus cavity) is caused by a viral infection in the upper respiratory tract, while in rare cases; it may be caused by a bacterial infection.

Hydrogen peroxide can help clear the effete matter from the sinus cavity and hence clear the congestion. Hydrogen peroxide has antibacterial properties. The oxygen released from hydrogen peroxide can help in eliminating the microbial infection. Rinsing your sinus cavity with hydrogen peroxide can prevent germs from re-infecting the damaged areas, thus giving your nasal membranes the time to heal. When the nasal membranes are healthy, they are more capable of resisting infection. It is cost-effective as compared to other treatment methods. One bottle of hydrogen peroxide can be used multiple times. Many other treatments, like steroidal nasal sprays, can be addictive and can cause the body to become tolerant. This means that you might progressively need a higher dosage as time passes to get the same effect. Hydrogen peroxide does not make your body dependent or addicted to it.

Place the mixture in a nasal spray container and spray it into your nose, blowing it back out after fifteen seconds. Spraying hydrogen peroxide into your nasal passages should help kill the infection. In addition, to help with a painful sinus infection, inhaling a few drops of peppermint oil will dissolve any sinus cavity quickly.

Ease a Sore Throat

You can use hydrogen peroxide in a couple of different ways to treat a sore throat. You can gargle a mixture of peroxide and warm boiled water, or you can dip a wool covered stick in 3% peroxide and coat your tonsils. Kindly be careful not to swallow hydrogen peroxide while adopting either of these remedies.

Appease Dry Skin

Hydrogen peroxide can be an excellent natural treatment for dry skin. When you apply half a pint of peroxide to your bath water, the added oxygen helps to rejuvenate your body and keeps your skin hydrated. The antiviral and antibacterial properties can also aid with various skin infections and conditions.

Clean and Disinfect Small Cuts

It can be applied directly to the wound to clean away any dead tissue. Doing this will help the wound to cease bleeding, and it's capable of clearing up infections and preventing new infections from coming up.

Using hydrogen peroxide on small cuts and wounds is one of the most popular uses of the miraculous chemical. To ensure you don't inhibit friendly bacteria from facilitating the healing process, you only want to apply it to the affected area once.

Treat Acne

Acne as a skin infection, if you suffer from acne that has become infected, try using hydrogen peroxide instead of antibacterial soap to help speed up the healing process. Applying it to acne on the skin will work in the same way as it does on wounds. It will not only clean the area, but it will also kill unwanted bacteria.

Just apply it to the infected area once to prevent destroying the good bacteria that your body requires to heal.

Treat Canker Sores

Hydrogen Peroxide can cure Canker sores or small shallow ulcers that form in your mouth. Combine it with some water and swish it around in your mouth for about thirty seconds, spit out and rinse with water and it will help you to get rid of a canker sore. It's important to remember to combine it with water since too much concentration can cause irritation and blistering.

Get Rid of Bad Breath with a Peroxide Mouth Rinse

Hydrogen peroxide is a miracle solution and has a multitude of uses. Mix equal parts hydrogen peroxide and water to make an effective bad-breath-fighting mouth wash. Swish the mixture in your mouth and spit, making sure not to swallow. Hydrogen peroxide is extremely effective at killing off bacteria in your mouth. Soaking your toothbrush in a bowl of hydrogen peroxide is also effective at killing the bacteria that builds up on your bristles. Just swishing with the chemical compound once a week can eliminate bad breath for seven days. Not to mention, it has teeth whitening properties. Watch how much you use, as overusing the mouthwash will end up killing the good bacteria that is in your mouth.

Battle Foot Fungus

If you're tired of the itching and burning that comes with athlete's foot and foot fungus, hydrogen peroxide's antifungal properties may be the perfect antidote.

Pour hydrogen peroxide directly onto the affected area. Note that it may sting, and it should bubble, especially if you have open wounds. Do this twice daily until the infection subsides.

Treat Nail Fungus

This is an oxidative therapy; essentially, it's the act of soaking the affected nail in hydrogen peroxide until the fungus gets destroyed due to the increased level of oxygen.

Obtain 3% hydrogen peroxide solution. Use a solution that is no more than a 3% concentration. A solution that is more than 3% is not as safe to use and may cause skin reactions.

Mix the hydrogen peroxide solution with an equal quantity of water or vinegar (if treating your feet).

Soak your infected nails in the solution for about 30 minutes each day. Continue the process for about a month without skipping any days, or until the fungus is totally grown out.

Treat Colds

It is important to begin treatment as soon as symptoms appear. If treatment is started promptly effectiveness seems to be in the 80% range.

You can mix it with kosher salt and baking soda to remove infections out of your nasal passage and put a couple of drops in your ears to kill any bacteria that have taken up residence in them.

Treat Ear Infections

Just a couple of drops of H2O2 can help you kill the bacteria that cause ear infections. Keep in mind that ear infections can get serious, so you may still want to visit the doctor if you are unable to cure your ear infection with this method.

Side note: Peroxide is not just used for human ear infections but also an ingredient of a good homemade ear cleaner for dogs.

Ear Wax Removal

If you have trouble hearing, it may be a result of a buildup of excess ear wax in your ears. Just like using hydrogen peroxide to get rid of ear infections, you can use it to remove ear wax. You'll hear better before you know it. Many solutions contain hydrogen peroxide. Hydrogen peroxide helps the wax bubble up and results in the wax becoming softer.

Lie down on your side. One ear should face up. Administer the instructed number of drops into your ear canal and fill it with fluid. Keep still for 5 minutes. Sit up after 5 minutes, and blot the outer ear with a tissue to absorb any liquid that comes out. Repeat this process for your other ear.

Treat Toothache

A toothache is a pain in and around the teeth and jaws. Tooth decay, an infection, loose or broken fillings, or receding gums can cause it.

If the pain lasts for more than 1 or 2 days, it is best to see a dentist immediately to have it treated.

Rinsing with a hydrogen peroxide solution is an effective antibacterial mouthwash, especially if a toothache is caused by an infection.

Hydrogen peroxide is dangerous if swallowed so great care must be taken when rinsing.

It should be mixed in equal parts of 3 percent hydrogen peroxide and water and swished in the mouth for about 30 seconds. After spitting it out, the mouth should be rinsed several times with plain water.

A hydrogen peroxide rinse must never be swallowed, and this remedy is not recommended for children.

Doing this will help significantly reduce the amount of pain you may be experiencing until you can get to a dentist. Avoid overusing this method to ensure you don't kill the good bacteria that live in your mouth.

Detoxifying Bath

Add ½ cup to 1 cup of 35% food grade peroxide to a bath-tub-full of water. Then get in and soak, preferably for 30 minutes or longer for a pleasant soak. It's perfect for helping you rid your body of all kinds of infections from the lower half of your body, including many STDs. You can also use salt or essential oils, or whatever sort of stuff you like to use in the bath, right along with the hydrogen peroxide. I've used Epsom salts, essential oils, and herbal infusions for my peroxide bath soaks.

This bath therapy not only does it detoxify the body and relieve pain, but it also seems to stop many infections quickly and help your body to regain balance. It has been shown in medical studies to relieve pain that does not respond to narcotic medicines.

For the bath, you will need 4-6 cups Epsom salt (magnesium sulfate), 32-64 fluid ounces of hydrogen peroxide (3%, as found in grocery stores), 2-4 Tbsp. of ginger (preferably fresh-grated and wrapped in a thin piece of cloth or a tea ball. An old piece of nylon hose also works well).

This and all bath therapies work best if you first dry brush the skin on your entire body. This removes any dead skin that may otherwise block the absorption of energy and nutrients. It also stimulates the blood and lymph fluids to rise to the skin to accept the healing effects of the bath. Do not use if you are pregnant.

Treating Yeast Infections

This is a common condition in women. It is characterized by intense itchiness of the vagina and discharge. Though medications can treat the infection, most often, it tends to interfere with a woman's normal life.

Hydrogen Peroxide has historically been great killer of candida, bacteria and viruses. Hydrogen peroxide is something that occurs naturally in the vagina and, in most cases works to prevent yeast infections by killing the main culprit, Candida albicans. Yeast infections occur when your body produces too much yeast, overwhelming the peroxide that occurs naturally in the body.

Hydrogen peroxide works by restoring the normal vaginal bacterial flora. It also restores the pH balance of the vagina, which could be another contributing factor to yeast infection.

Hydrogen peroxide also helps remove clue cells. These are cells on the vaginal skin that are covered with the infection-causing microbes.

In a healthy vagina, the good bacteria (lactobacillus) produce lactic acid and hydrogen peroxide. These two create an acidic and protective environment, thereby preventing the infection. Using hydrogen peroxide to treat a vaginal yeast infection is simple. But strongly recommend you use it in addition to your prescribed medications after consulting your doctor.

Get 2 cups of hydrogen peroxide, Add the hydrogen peroxide to a tub half-filled with water. Soak in it for about 30 minutes. You can do this once daily.

Teeth Whitener

Tooth whitening has become more popular in recent years as more products come onto the market. But many of these products can be quite expensive, leading people to look for cheaper remedies.

The most affordable way to whiten teeth at home (and the remedy supported by the most significant body of research) is the main ingredient from most tooth-whitening products: hydrogen peroxide.

To keep your smile looking bright, swish hydrogen peroxide around in your mouth for at least thirty seconds, once a week.

Doing this will not only assist in whitening your teeth, but it will also kill the bacteria that causes bad breath. Along with being a germicidal agent, it also acts as a bleaching agent.

Use as a Toothpaste

To create all-natural toothpaste, void of the artificial ingredients that are common in the name brand tubes of toothpaste, simply mix a small amount of baking soda and hydrogen peroxide and use to brush your teeth.

Making this kind of paste is not only easy, but it also doesn't contain any harsh, artificial chemicals. Peroxide also serves as an excellent DIY denture cleaner.

Disinfect Toothbrush

How do you put your toothbrush away after using it? If you're like most people, you probably just rinse, shake, and put it in the medicine cabinet. However, did you know that moist places are a perfect home for bacteria? This means that the germs and bacteria you brushed away on your toothbrush stay there until you brush again. How do we keep our toothbrush from leftover or new bacteria?

Pour hydrogen peroxide into a container (enough to soak the toothbrush's head). Leave your toothbrush in the hydrogen peroxide for at least 5 minutes. Thoroughly rinse your toothbrush to get rid of the hydrogen peroxide taste. Shake off any additional moisture. Place your toothbrush in a dry spot, away from other toothbrushes and moisture. Safely pour hydrogen peroxide down the sink. Repeat once a week.

Precautions to take don't use a cover for your brush's head (prevents your toothbrush from drying). Don't put your toothbrush in a closed container. Keep hydrogen peroxide away from the sun for longer shelf life. Replace your toothbrush every 3 months

Treatment for Gum Disease

Because of its antibacterial properties, hydrogen peroxide may help treat gum disease.

Plaque that forms on the teeth contains a slimy film of bacteria called a biofilm. Hydrogen peroxide releases oxygen that helps destroy the bacteria. One advantage of gargling with a hydrogen peroxide solution is it can reach the back of the mouth and spots that may be hard to reach with dental floss.

Use a 3% concentration of hydrogen peroxide. Anything stronger is likely to cause irritation. Mix two parts water with one part hydrogen peroxide. Gargle, swishing the solution all around the mouth. Tilt the head back and continue gargling for 30 seconds. Spit the solution out. The hydrogen peroxide may cause some foaming in the mouth, which is normal. To avoid irritating the gums, consider limiting use to a few times a week.

Beauty Used of Hydrogen Peroxide

Use as Deodorant

Most deodorants on the market today contain aluminum, which may deter you from wanting to smear it into your skin. And, there are some natural deodorants on the market that actually work, but they can be pretty expensive. So, the next logical step is to create a natural deodorant of your own. You can do this using hydrogen peroxide and baking soda.

Add one-part water to two-part hydrogen peroxide in a small spray bottle and shake lightly to combine. Spritz the solution onto your underarm area and dab a bit of baking soda on afterwards. This will work to prevent odors, but it does not work as an antiperspirant, which means you may still sweat, it just won't smell as bad.

Mixing hydrogen peroxide with dish soap at a ratio of 1:2, you create an effective deodorant. Apply the mixture to your underarms, leaving it in place for 30 minutes, and then rinse it off.

Doing so can help you stay dry and odor-free for up to 24 hours. While you may not want to use this procedure every day, because dish soap is very sticky, it may work well in a pinch.

Clean Makeup Brushes

Using hydrogen peroxide to clean makeup brushes makes the painful process easier. All you need is 1 part 3% hydrogen peroxide and 1 part water.

Mix 3% peroxide with water and soak your brushes for five minutes, followed by rinsing the brushes clean. For squeaky clean brushes, repeat this process once a week.

Whiten Your Nails

Just like it can whiten your teeth, hydrogen peroxide is an excellent way to whiten your nails. Nails can face issues like yellowing and staining due factors like poor diet and using dark nail polishes for a longer period. Stained nails can easily be corrected/whitened using a simple home ingredient. Add 3% hydrogen peroxide and equal quantity of water in a bowl. Stir and soak your nails in it for 15 minutes. Gently brush your nails with a soft and clean toothbrush and follow with a good moisturizer. Do this once daily (if required) until you are satisfied with the results.

Cover Darker Roots

If you bleach your hair blonde, you may get frustrated when your roots start to show in between hair appointments. You can remedy this situation by bleaching hair some hydrogen peroxide to your roots and letting it bleach for half an hour before rinsing it out.

If you do this often enough it can help conceal your dark roots before your next hair appointment.

Lighten the Hair

If you want to subtly lighten or dye your hair over a period, without resorting to coloring your hair, hydrogen peroxide is a great alternative.

To employ this method, mix peroxide with equal parts water and place it in a spray bottle. Spray your hair with the solution and comb through your hair to help distribute the mixture. Allow it to dry. Doing this on a regular basis will gradually add blonde highlights to your hair.

Soften Corns and Calluses on Your Feet

Corns and calluses can make moving your foot not just uncomfortable, but even painful if not treated.

Hydrogen peroxide is a great natural agent that can significantly soften those pesky corns and calluses.

Simply mix one cup of the peroxide with ½ a cup of water in a bowl, stir well, and let sit for five minutes. Soak the affected foot for fifteen minutes.

Remove your foot from the solution, rinse it with clean water, and dry it thoroughly. Continue doing this several times a week for three weeks to get permanent relief.

House Cleaning Uses of Hydrogen Peroxide

The antibacterial properties make hydrogen peroxide suitable for disinfecting the different surfaces around your house. Cleaning your home with it not only helps prevent the members of your home from becoming sick, but it's also ideal to avoid the disease from spreading.

Disinfecting Countertops

You can use hydrogen peroxide to disinfect your bathroom and kitchen countertops and every other hard surface where germs and bacteria can be.

Simply mix it with equal parts water and put it in a spray bottle. Spray down your surfaces and use a sponge to wipe them down.

Whiten Grout

Hydrogen peroxide is a natural alternative to bleach that brightens and eliminates germs. Plus it is non-toxic and decomposes into water and oxygen. The collection of dust and dirt on your grout can quickly make it look dingy and dirty, and nothing is worse than dirty grout. To make the best DIY grout cleaner, and bring it back to its original white, simply spray hydrogen peroxide onto dry grout and let it sit for several hours.

Once you've given it enough time to penetrate the dirt and grime that has accumulated, come back with soapy water and a toothbrush and vigorously scrub the grout. After drying it off, the grout should look clean, white, and new.

Cleaning the Mirrors

Most of the commercial cleaners you use on your mirrors leave unsightly stains, no matter how hard you try to stop them. Hydrogen peroxide has been shown to be a perfect no-strip cleaner for mirrors. Just spray the solvent onto your mirrors and wipe it off with a paper towel. A bonus for using peroxide to disinfect your mirrors: it destroys the germs of the bathroom that have accumulated on the window.

Clean Toilet

Do you need to know how to clean a toilet? Disinfecting your toilet bowl has never been easier.

As part of a homemade toilet cleaner, pour four ounces of a bottle of hydrogen peroxide into your toilet and let it stand for twenty minutes.

Come back and scrub out the toilet with your toilet brush, and flush. You can also douse your toilet brush with the peroxide to disinfect it and keep it sanitary and clean.

Get rid of a clogged toilet, too, with some hydrogen peroxide, vinegar, and baking soda. The DIY way is almost always the best solution!

If you have accumulated some unwanted hard water stains, peroxide can also help in this situation. How to clean toilet bowl stains involves adding some peroxide to the bowl, scrubbing with the toilet brush, and letting the solution sit for a while.

Overnight soaking offers the best results. It may be necessary to repeat the process several times to completely eliminate the stains.

Clean Bathroom Tiles

The tiles in your bathroom can become extremely disgusting due to the build-up of soap dirt and stains, and you can use hydrogen peroxide to brighten the tiles while destroying germs and mold and mildew that have begun to form.

Mix it with flour to form a paste and apply it directly to the tiles. Cover the area with plastic wrap and let the mixture stand overnight. The next morning, you simply have to rinse the tiles until they become clean.

Peroxide is such a powerful bathroom cleaner, it can even be used to get rid of rust stains in your in your toilet and tub.

Kills Mold

Eliminate mold from the bathroom and any other areas of your home, by treating it with full-strength hydrogen peroxide. Just apply it with a rag or a spray bottle, and let it sit for 30 minutes. Then, come back and clean the area.

Hydrogen peroxide will kill mold, but it won't eliminate mold stains. You'll need to do a deep cleaning afterwards to make that happen.

Remove Stains from Marble

Unsealed marble is prone to staining (even water can stain it). Address stains as soon as you notice them by making a paste of flour and hydrogen peroxide, and applying it directly to the stained surface. Cover the area with plastic wrap, to keep the paste from drying out, and let it sit overnight. Then, clean up the paste in the morning, and the stain should be gone, or at least greatly lightened. Repeat the process, if needed.

Consider sealing your marble once you get it cleaned, to protect it from future stains. It only takes a couple minutes to do. Be sure to test this stain solution in an inconspicuous area the first time you use it.

Cleaning Windows

Use hydrogen peroxide to clean your windows without having to worry about harmful chemicals. 3/4 cup hydrogen peroxide, A couple of drops of scented dish soap and Water

Take one of your spray bottles and add hydrogen peroxide, dish soap, and water. Apply the mixture to windows and allow it to sit for several minutes to help loosen the dirt, oils, and grime that has accumulated on the surface of the windows.

Then wipe the window down with a clean paper towel. If the windows still have some residue on them, you can repeat the process.

Water Sanitation

If your well water smells like rotten-eggs, you are not alone. Well water odor is a common problem and many homeowners battle stinky well water. Rotten-egg water not only has an objectionable odor, but in high concentrations may be dangerous to your health, and is corrosive to plumbing, fixtures and appliances.

Water containing hydrogen sulfide gas ("H2S"), has a unique "rotten egg" odor, which is often present in both hot and cold, but may become more pronounced from the hot water. This kind of water can discolor coffee, tea and other beverages, and alter the appearance as well as taste of cooked food.

Water containing H2S can corrode piping materials, such as copper, brass, steel and iron as well as exposed metallic components inside dishwashers and appliances tarnishing the surfaces a black color. Hydrogen sulfide can also quickly foul and ruin water softeners and filter systems.

Hydrogen Peroxide is better in treating water; it works faster than chlorine, so often no contact tank is required. Unlike chlorine will not leave a chemical residual in the water. Peroxide works over a wider pH range.

Like chlorine, hydrogen peroxide is a strong oxidizer and can quickly eliminate the odors. Unlike chlorine however, hydrogen peroxide leaves behind no trace of chemical by-products. When hydrogen peroxide is injected into water, a large amount of dissolved oxygen is released and a strong oxidizing effect takes place. Odors are eliminated, microorganisms are destroyed, and tannins can be oxidized.

Clean Children's Toys

Children, in particular infants and toddlers, tend to stick everything in their mouths, leaving them crawling with germs and bacteria. As a result, your child can end up becoming sick.

Clean kids' toys and play areas. Hydrogen peroxide is a safe cleaner to use around kids, or anyone with respiratory problems, because it's not a lung irritant. Spray toys, toy boxes, doorknobs, and anything else your kids touch on a regular basis.

Cleaning Humidifier or Dehumidifier

Because of the constant flow of moisture through these devices, they tend to accumulate mold.

To keep this from getting out of control and becoming a sanitation issue, you can run a mixture of water and hydrogen peroxide through the device to kill the mold that has accumulated inside. If you want to continue to process clean air, it's important to clean your humidifiers regularly.

Kitchen Uses of Hydrogen Peroxide

When used as an antibacterial and germicidal agent, hydrogen peroxide is great for cleaning just about everything around your house. It's also convenient to use in the kitchen. There are numerous specific applications for the compound that can help you keep your kitchen clean and free of germs.

Clean Your Cutting Boards

Cutting boards are vulnerable to the accumulation of harmful germs and bacteria. By using your cutting board, you can clean it with fresh water and then spray it with hydrogen peroxide to take care of the germs so they can find their way to other foods while you are preparing your utensils.

Add It to Your Dishwasher

If you find that your dishes are not as sparkling clean as you want them to be when you run them through the dishwasher, you can use hydrogen peroxide to improve the efficiency of your dishwasher.

Add a couple of ounces of peroxide to your dish detergent to help your dishwasher do a better job. It helps and is also a great way to clean a dishwasher regularly. You can also add some to your regular dish soap to give it a boost in killing germs.

Disinfect the Inside of Your Cooler with Peroxide

Coolers tend to have the same problem with lunch boxes. After a summer of continuous use, they continue to be ignored, resulting in a build-up of food residues. To help you clean them and keep your entire family safe, simply wipe them off like a lunch box.

Sanitize Your Reusable Bags

Many people are starting to use reusable shopping bags when they head to the grocery store, which is an excellent way to eliminate waste and protect the environment. Just like with your kid's lunchboxes and coolers, these bags need to be disinfected from time to time.

To properly clean your reusable shopping bags, turn the bags inside out and spray the fabric with hydrogen peroxide. Not only with this disinfect the bag, but it will help to eliminate any lingering odors from the food.

Removes Stubborn Caked-On Food

If you're struggling to extract stubborn cake-on food from your pots and pans, hydrogen peroxide will help. Only mix it with some baking soda to form a paste and rub it into a sore spot and let it sit for a few minutes.

Use warm water to scrub to problematic stain away. The baking soda cleans as an abrasive, while the peroxide assists in breaking up the particles.

Disinfect Your Sponges and Dishrags

The more you use your sponges and dishrags, the more germs and bacteria they will pick up, and when they sit around, the bacteria and germs can multiply and an alarming rate.

To prevent this from happening and kill germs and bacteria, soak them in hydrogen peroxide, or even spray them with a solution while they're sitting in the sink. Using peroxide to clean your sponges and dishrags will not only keep you free from dangerous germs, but will prolong the life of your sponges.

Clean Your Fruits and Vegetables

Hydrogen peroxide works great for cleaning your fruits and vegetables of harmful pesticides. There are several ways to accomplish this.

Next, you should spray some food-grade peroxide on them and let them sit down for a few minutes before rinsing and leaving them to dry. You may also apply a little vinegar to another spray bottle and mix it with peroxide. They're both working together to detoxify your food.

Keeping Fruits and Vegetables Fresh

Hydrogen peroxide can extend the life of your fresh vegetables and fruit. With a sink full of water, apply a quarter cup of hydrogen peroxide in the food grade and soak in it for 20 minutes.

After they have soaked, rinse and dry them. Peroxide eliminates the contaminants that have accumulated during the growing cycle and preserves freshness.

Keeping Salad Fresh

Salads seem to wilt very easily. If you want to keep your salad fresh for longer, you can mix two tablespoons of peroxide with one cup of water and sprinkle it over your salad. Make sure you use peroxide of the food grade and dilute the peroxide properly.

Cleaning the Fridge

If your fridge has started to smell a bit funky, you can use hydrogen peroxide to get rid of the unpleasant odors, while disinfecting the surfaces. Wipe down the shelves and the insides of the fridge with peroxide to get rid of ugly food stains, kill germs, and neutralize many of the odors. To take care of the rest of the odors, add a box of open baking soda to your fridge.

Grow Mushrooms in Refrigerator

You can use hydrogen peroxide to grow oyster mushrooms in your refrigerator. The process takes about six months, from start to finish, but will result in a ton of free mushrooms.

Watch this video on how to grow mushrooms in your refrigerator, an astonishing way to use peroxide.

Disinfect Kid's Lunchboxes

How often do you wash out your child's lunchbox? Chances are not very often, which can result in it getting nasty with the buildup of overlooked food residue.

To keep their lunch box clean and free from germs and bacteria, spray it with hydrogen peroxide at the end of the week. Let it sit for a few minutes before rinsing with clean water and wiping it down.

Making sure to disinfect your children's lunchboxes on a regular basis to help keep them healthy.

Hydrogen Peroxide usage in the Laundry Room

Are your white towels and clothing looking just a little bit dingy these days? Or smelling less than pleasant? Hydrogen peroxide to the rescue! Just add one cup of 3 percent hydrogen peroxide solution (it's probably the kind you have already, but be sure to check) to your washing machine before you add the clothing or water.

Hydrogen peroxide makes a great substitute for bleach, especially in a pinch, but just makes sure to either test the fabrics first or only use it on whites because it can stain dark fabrics. Hydrogen peroxide is also a more environmentally friendly product than bleach, so you can feel good about using it. Soak the fabrics for about 30 minutes to pull the unsightly yellowing from your whites to make them look cleaner and feel fresher.

However, it is important to note that you don't need to go overboard and use both hydrogen peroxide and bleach at the same time. Your clothing won't be any cleaner. This is because the sodium hypochlorite in the chlorine bleach will overpower the hydrogen peroxide, essentially turning it into water.

Peroxide, oxygen bleach, vinegar, and baking soda can all help remove mildew from clothes, as well.

If you left wet laundry in the machine overnight accidentally or put wet clothes in the dryer without turning it on, you likely have mold and mildew that has formed on clothing. Rewash the clothes with one of the previously mentioned cleaners to get rid of that unsightly and smelly mold.

Brighten Curtains and Table Cloths

If your white curtains and tablecloths have turned yellow and rusty, you can clean the yellow areas with some hydrogen peroxide to give new life to your linens and curtains. You can also put a little hydrogen peroxide in the washing machine to brighten them and make them look new.

Wash Your Shower Curtains

Your shower curtains love to collect soap scum and mildew like they are going out of style. To kill the mildew and remove tough soap scum from your shower curtain, use hydrogen peroxide.

If your shower curtain can go in the washing machine, run it through the rinse cycle with some hydrogen peroxide, or you can wash it by hand, by spraying it down with the peroxide and scrubbing it down with a sponge and rinsing with fresh water.

Remove Tough Stains from White Clothing

Several types of stains are particularly tricky to get rid of, like blood stains or sweat stains that form in the armpits of shirts. All you need is 2 parts hydrogen peroxide and 1 part detergent

You can use a mixture of two parts hydrogen peroxide and one part detergent to deal with these hard to remove stains. Place the solution directly onto the stains and let sit.

Then run your clothes through a cycle in the washing machine and watch them vanish. Be sure you just use this procedure for white colored clothes, because the peroxide can bleach dark or patterned fabrics.

Clean Rugs, Carpet and Mattress

You can spray hydrogen peroxide on your rugs, carpets or mattresses to avoid dirt or urine stains and unsightly food stains. Also make sure you do this with light colored fabrics, because you could end up bleaching dark colored fabrics, leaving fresh, hideous patches instead. We cover different cleaning recipes for our tips on how to clean a mattress.

If you make your own homemade carpet shampoo, please make sure you don't overuse hydrogen peroxide. To see if this will bleach your rug or carpet; test it on an inconspicuous spot, like inside your closet or under an item of furniture.

Remove Odors from Clothes and Carpet

If your clothes, upholstery or carpet smell a bit musty, you can use hydrogen peroxide to eliminate the foul smelling odor and make your clothes smell fresh.

Remove odors from your clothes by mixing peroxide with white vinegar and adding it to your wash. Make sure you only do this with your light colored clothing.

In addition to getting rid of any carpet or upholstery smells a mixture of hydrogen peroxide, baking soda, and liquid dish soap works best. To get cat urine smell out of carpet or upholstery spray it on and let it dry. When you vacuum the residue all smells will be gone.

Hydrogen Peroxide usage in Gardening

Increase Plant Growth with Hydrogen Peroxide

Have you ever seen how rainwater makes your plants grow faster? Hydrogen peroxide for plants is naturally present in the rain. You can soak the seeds in a solution of one ounce of peroxide for every two cups of water to simulate rain and help improve the growth of your plants.

Soak the seed overnight, then plant as usual. To improve the health of your current plants, spray them with a solution of 1-part peroxide to 32-part water.

It can also help to protect your plants from harmful sun damage. Plants use a chemical that naturally occurs as a by-product of photosynthesis to regulate how their cells respond to varying levels of light.

Get Rid of Weeds

If you're sick of keeping pesky weeds out of your lawn and garden, hydrogen peroxide is an outstanding Do it yourself weed killer. You only have to mix one ounce of 3% peroxide with one quarter of water and spray it on the weeds. Let stand for about 15 minutes, then rinse with water.

Cleaning Compost Buckets

While compost buckets are great for the environment, they tend to harbor harmful germs and bacteria and can begin to smell atrocious.

To keep it from developing an unbearable stink and becoming gross too quickly, add an inch of 3 percent hydrogen peroxide into the bottom of the bucket to clean it out and start off right. As you add food to the bucket, the peroxide allows you to keep it in your kitchen for a bit longer with quite a bit less stench.

Eliminate Algae from Your Aquarium

Home aquariums not only add beauty to your home décor but can give you therapeutic benefits as well. The only downside is cleaning the fish tanks, particularly when algae begin to accumulate.

To clean your fish tank, safely and efficiently, without causing harm to the inhabitants, is to use hydrogen peroxide. To keep your fish and plants from being hurt, you want to only use about 60 milliliters of three percent peroxide per 66 gallons of water.

Slowly apply the peroxide to the tank with a syringe or dropper for five minutes. If you can, try adding it directly to the algae. It will react with the algae, destroy it, and then dilute it.

Hydrogen Peroxide for Animal and Pet Care

Kill Mites

While mites or spider mites may not be harmful to humans, they can be a pain if you find them in your home. To get rid of them without contaminating your house or yard with toxic chemicals, just spray some hydrogen peroxide wherever you find them.

Help Transport Fish

If you transport fish in a tank, adding hydrogen peroxide to the water will help keep your fish more secure and healthier during transport. You want to use the little white tablets that dissolve in water for a more controlled release of oxygen.

Treat Animal Wounds

You may use hydrogen peroxide to treat wounds in animals, just as you would treat your wounds. Squeezing it gently on the wound will help to remove any dead tissue and destroy any bacteria that might be in the wound.

Induce Vomiting to Save Your Pet's Life

You can use the 3% peroxide to help induce vomiting if your pet has ingested something toxic. Use for cats, dogs, ferrets, and pigs. Do not use this method on rodents, rabbits, horses, squirrels or birds, or ruminant animals. Before giving peroxide to your pet, try and get them to eat something, increasing their likelihood of vomiting.

If they refuse to eat anything, use a syringe to squirt 1 millimeter of peroxide per pound of weight in the back of the animal's mouth. Your pet will start vomiting within 15 minutes. If it doesn't work after a second attempt, take your pet to the vet.

Remove Skunk Odors

Mixing dish soap, baking soda, and hydrogen peroxide is a good way to get rid of skunk odor. It works because the oxygen molecules help to neutralize the scent by bonding to the thiols.

Altering the chemical makeup contributes to eliminating the stench quickly. Skunks also do not like the smell of hydrogen peroxide so the liquid makes a natural skunk repellent, too.

Hydrogen Peroxide Side Effects

While hydrogen peroxide is a natural chemical compound, it can cause severe side effects if it is not properly used or ingested. If swallowed, undiluted and high concentrations of the chemical can cause the following side effects:

- Vomiting
- Mouth, throat, and stomach burns
- Stomach bleeding
- Gastrointestinal issues
- Stomach ulcers
- Rupture of the colon

- Stoke
- Brain swelling
- Death

When using hydrogen peroxide for medicinal purposes, please be careful and follow the instructions carefully.

Just use the lowest peroxide grade, 3%, that you can find in the pharmaceutical section of your local grocery store. Higher grades of chemicals, known as food grades, can be particularly dangerous and should be avoided at all costs.

How and Where to Buy Hydrogen Peroxide

From your local supermarket or drugstore, you can buy 3% hydrogen peroxide. Most of the chemical grades can also be ordered online from locations like amazon.

61+ AMAZING USES AND BENEFITS OF HYDROGEN PEROXIDE
BY ERIC GOLDINGER

WARNING

Hydrogen peroxide functions very well at present and in many ways to overcome health issues, but you do not drink it. Hydrogen peroxide is prescribed by natural medicine practitioners for all kinds of circumstances: it is all about flu and cancer. The aim is to create an oxygen-rich atmosphere in which bacteria cannot survive by consuming hydrogen peroxide on a daily basis. Your body naturally produces hydrogen peroxide itself as part of your immune response. So the thought says, "Why don't you make more if it works?"

So, why are you not supposed to do that? Of course, your immune system generates hydrogen peroxide, but it does so in such a manner that hydrogen peroxide is unable to harm other cells in your body. It's contained in a phagosome compartment. When you ingest hydrogen peroxide, it is safe and therefore can cause oxidative stress to harm all tissues in your body. This can be one of the cancer triggers in fact. This could actually make things worse by orally taking H2O2. Furthermore, elevated doses can trigger oral vesicles, abdominal pain, diarrhea and vomiting even at a concentration of 3 percent. Taking it intravenously is just as bad.

Although oral hydrogen peroxide cannot be used to cure health conditions, minor injuries, ear infections, colds, sinus infections, toothaches, fungal infections, etc. are very well handled. There are many uses for beauty and hygiene, and use at home, particularly in the kitchen, is a great cleaning and disinfecting agent. Hydrogen peroxide is so unbelievable that in a tough place you can even use it to save a pet's life.

www.ingramcontent.com/pod-product-compliance
Lightning Source LLC
Chambersburg PA
CBHW050252220526
45465CB00002B/645